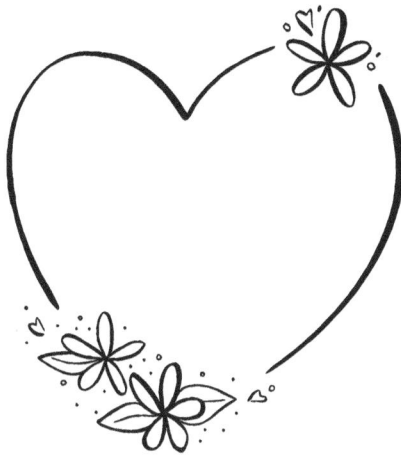

RESTORED
TO
WHOLENESS

ALSO BY THE AUTHOR

RISING FROM THE FIRE

SURRENDERING TO WHO YOU ARE

FREE YOUR SOUL

THE HARMONY WITHIN

THE WISDOM WITHIN

THE HOME WITHIN

LIFE ON FIRE JOURNAL

Please scan the link above to view all the titles currently available by this author. Thank you.

MURIEL OKUBO

Doctor of Asian Medicine

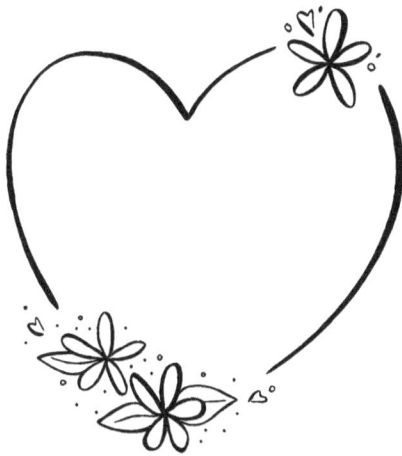

RESTORED TO WHOLENESS

Inspirational Reflections on Harnessing Strength
in Adversity and Embracing the Power to Heal

Hardcover ISBN: 978-1-998695-03-4
Paperback ISBN: 978-1-998695-02-7
EBOOK ISBN: 978-1-998695-04-1

To the divine souls who helped me in my time of need. Thank you.

Welcome Friend,

When facing your humanity, steady, encouraging support is your lifeline in adverse times. Hence, many poems emphasize repetition, repeatedly reminding you of your power. Consistency and persistence are crucial to overcoming the inevitable dips and hurdles on the road to success and recovery. Repetition and positive reinforcement are your friends.

TABLE OF CONTENTS

INTRODUCTION

INTRODUCTION

Over my career as a Doctor of Asian Medicine, I've witnessed many people facing complex challenges and adversities. I have approached each patient with a healing mindset. Our health and healing capacity is unlimited when we're open to possibilities. This mindset leaves room for miracles and makes us a magnet for wisdom beyond the limits of our consciousness. These principles can open doors to our healing and restoration.

When we focus on the best possible outcomes, our energy can move towards achieving them, leaving no time to dwell on potential adverse outcomes or worst-case scenarios. This approach is essential for restoring our health and wellness beyond what our physical senses may relay.

These principles were not just theories to me; they were my lifeline during a long season that challenged me physically, mentally, emotionally, and spiritually. By God's grace, I'm here on the other side.

I understood a new level of perseverance, patience, compassion, and love for myself.

Love, in its purest form, became my healer and restorer, offering me comfort, wisdom, and reassurance in a dark season. It was the foundation for everything I needed and a guiding light that led to my healing.

We're sacred beings who often forget the truth of who we are and the vastness of everything we've been given. Adversity will call us to harness a strength we never knew was available.

After my experience, I wrote these verses to process and share what I learned from my healing. It also includes my perspective from years of treating people over my career. Writing in this form turns the most heart-wrenching experiences into beauty, which is how I choose to digest life. I hope these verses resonate with the shared humanity of readers facing their own struggles.

As we become more spiritually conscious, let's have compassion for everyone facing their unique battles. Without empathy, a willingness to understand, and a growth consciousness, we hinder our ability to function and thrive fully as individuals and as a society. Although our afflictions may differ, our consciousness can bridge and connect us with power, love, and strength.

Earth school requires much of us, and I hope health and wellness become standard practice everywhere.

This book shares the core energy of my restoration to wholeness. It's about embracing my power to heal and honouring the life I've been gifted. May it inspire your health journey. My experiences are embedded in these verses, and I hope healing touches your heart, body, mind, spirit, and soul. Each piece extends from my heart to yours.

Let these words remind you of the strength and perseverance you possess, especially in times of challenge and adversity. Believe in the power of your healing. Be inspired by the fact that change is always possible for the better and for your restoration. You have the strength within you to overcome, and you're more resilient than you may realize.

You're not alone. Don't give up wherever you are and whatever you may be facing. Hold onto the divine inner power and let your soul lead you to the necessary answers and miracles. Health is indeed wealth.

Thank you for choosing this book and spending your time with me.

HARNESSING YOUR ENERGY

When faced with our own humanity,
our perception of the world changes.
We learn what it is to fight for our lives.
Our soul knows what it takes to light the fire
after it's been extinguished.
How much starter fluid
do we need to ignite it?
What will it take to burn again?
Will it come from inspiration?
Love, patience, and diligence
will put us on the path of restoration.
Our heart and spirit will harness
the wisdom and knowledge we need,
revealing to us
supernatural cures, miracles, and treasures.
This is how we survive.
This is how we thrive.

ONE TRUTH

Our divine nature was made to heal.
We're incredible beings who
have inherent healing powers.
The more I seek,
the more I realize
nature's principles are straightforward.
The body will strive for balance
when there is an imbalance.
Every disease,
every disorder—
it's the same.
When I hear people saying
something is incurable,
is it because we don't yet have the cure,
or because we lack the knowledge,
or is it, indeed,
something we must contend with?
There is very little I believe is incurable—
despite our exposure to more pressures
and toxins than ever before.
As long as we live,
we must strive to obtain balance.

Miracles don't resonate
with lies or ignorance,
but with the truth of who we are.
When someone heals,
be grateful and happy
we heard their story.
One day,
this may grow our faith
and give us the conviction
to revive us from something
someone says is incurable
or non-recoverable.

SIGNALS

Life is a huge opportunity
to learn about ourselves.
It's a giant game of hot and cold.
We all have goals in life,
and what the world shows us,
will reveal if we're growing closer to our desires,
or if we're moving further away from them.
Our consciousness is vast,
and, sometimes,
it takes time to discover the truth.
It's this disconnect from the truth
that makes it seem our goals
are happening slowly.
Life is a feedback game,
and everything holds meaningful
and useful information.
Everything has been an opportunity
to increase our awareness
and understanding
of our purpose in this life.
For now,
our purpose is to recognize
if we're growing hotter or colder,
and to move ourselves in a better direction—

muriel okubo
8

if we inch closer to peace and joy,
then we're on the right track.
Pain signals are helpful, too.
They tell us where we hold energy in our system
and what needs to move or be released.
We need to do the things that support us
to move forward with the truth
and release the things
that take us away from the truth.

SHERLOCK HOLMES

The body is constantly seeking balance.
It has specific needs,
and it'll compensate for a long time.
It'll make do with what it's given
until it hits its breaking point.
And sometimes,
when the body
has a deluge of trouble thrown its way,
it will manage what it can
and shut down what it can't.
Along the way,
it'll give us signs of what it needs,
and, if not received,
it'll speak louder.
If severely out of balance,
it'll scream
and demand we take notice.
The body is good at adapting,
we often must become
Sherlock Holmes
to investigate the issues.
Often, it's this delicate balance—
too much,
too little,

what's just right?
As we become friends
with Sherlock Holmes inside ourselves—
the one in each of us;
that kind, soft, intelligent seeker
who is unassuming but wise
and has made it their mission
to keep us alive.

THE REALITY OF LOVE

True love is a blessing.
It's self-sacrificing
when it isn't easy.
It says,
"I'll be there for you."
And being there—
even when it's not convenient.
It's life-giving
when it feels like
we're drowning in quicksand.

HOLISTIC

All tragedies have the ability
to restore us to wholeness—
to remind us of why we came here,
to remind us of what love means,
to remind us that we can change our lives.
Everything can shift us
into our wholeness.
Frustration can lead to new growth.
Bitterness can soften our hearts again.
Worry can help us seek solid truth.
Sadness can inspire new ideas.
Fear can jolt us to take responsibility.

CHOICE

There are many ways to solve a problem.
Some methods are better than others.
What works for one
may be different from
what works for another.
What's apparent to one
may not be meaningful to another.
This is how it is.
Wisdom gives us the path
that best fits each of us individually.
We're all discovering the truth of who we are,
yet it's only in transparency
that we can solve the puzzle
that is us.

ENERGY MOVES

We all face challenges—
our own unique set of things to overcome.
There are many variables
that can cause disease
and many that help us
to overcome it.
Our energy is the most important
resource we have.
When we move energy
to where it needs to be,
and when we take it away
from an area of excess,
we create an environment of mutual support.
In freedom, we create movement.
Health abounds
with a free flow of energy.
This is the balance of life.

STRENGTH

On one of my darkest days,
a friend told me
to focus on the divine strength inside me.
Those words helped me through days
when I felt my world caving in.
I reminded myself
I have everything I need.
Sometimes,
when overwhelmed,
we desperately seek
an anchor of peace.
I have discovered
peace can only be found within.
It's a continual process
of returning to the light within myself
when the world is dark.

RESPECT YOURSELF

When the world
is confusing and conflicting,
default to the truth that bubbles within.
Intuition saves us from potential pitfalls—
telling us to back away,
double-check,
reconsider,
and take our time.
Fear tells us we're being silly,
that we must do it now,
that everyone else knows better,
that we can't wait.
There is a divine voice inside us,
that loves us,
and will speak to us.
Trust that voice
even if no one else does.
It'll feel peaceful
and gracious.
It can save our lives.

NOTHING COMPARES

This life is often
one of inconsistency,
incongruence, and dissonance.
The power of love
bridges this disorder.
Love clears confusion—
it's truthful,
wise,
compassionate,
kind,
and it never ceases.
This is the only thing
that keeps humanity alive
and puts everything in our favour.

PRINCIPLES

What I love about nature,
is that it seeks to work in harmony with us.
With this perspective,
I understand the opportunity to collaborate.
Control takes away life,
whereas freedom gives life.
With these principles,
I learned
true medicine should
support and free me.

IN THE THICK OF IT

When the weather is perfect and beautiful,
sunshine beams down on you.
Just for a moment,
you wish you could experience it the way,
your whole self would.
What would it be like
to feel like yourself
and the world to be a mirror of wellness?
You used to dream of those days,
put a smile on your face,
and believe you were okay.
On challenging days,
you disguised it well.
Only the people closest to you
knew you were falling apart.
When you're in harsh times,
trust is essential.
Everything can break you
when you're fragile.
You learned this is normal,
and you must hold hands
with discernment.
People who don't know you—

don't know your heart
and will judge you
when you're not yourself.
It's the love of people who know your soul,
who can give you the breath of life
when you need to be reminded
of who you are
and make space for you
to come back to yourself.

THE FIRE OF FAITH

I have always had great faith
in the healing abilities of our bodies.
I've witnessed it time and time again.
I've seen it in patients' lives
and in my own.
I know love and truth
are the antidotes to all illnesses.
I also know there's a song
in each of us
needing to be sung.

Sometimes, we're confronted
by everything that seems
to be the opposite
of love and truth—
but remember,
from someone who has witnessed the truth,
to ignore those who have lost their light,
and let your flame ignite from
the part of you that
knows you're a miracle of life.
Lean on your light
when you feel the darkness creep in.

If it's in your heart—
something you must sing,
do, be, or create in this life,
keep going.
Use it as a reminder
you're not meant to give up.
Wherever you are today,
let the truth move you,
and know that love can heal you.
Use everything you have
to fight for your life.
Keep going when you don't feel
like things are changing as quickly
as you would like—
what you must do,
only *you* can do.
Keep going,
my friend.

JUST AS YOU ARE

When we're vulnerable,
it's like we expose the underbelly of a turtle.
It's here we can be killed,
but it's also here we can be
tickled with delight.
Being strong has taught us
the vulnerability of being soft.
Being soft has taught us
the power of discovering our strength.
We can be both—
simultaneously
and exclusively.
Both are necessary
and welcome
in the wholeness that is us.

THE TRUTH OF LOVE

True love has taught me
that love doesn't leave
when uncomfortable.
It embraces us when we're powerless.
It forgives us when we're human.
It's patient when we're blind.
It's kind when we don't deserve it.
It's giving when we don't have anything.
It's humble when we're desperate.
It's peaceful when challenged.
It's honourable when no one sees.
It gives shelter from storms.
It trusts when faced with adversity.
It doesn't give up,
and it takes the long haul.

WORD POWER

I'm careful with my words.
I know they hold great power.
I never will use my words to hurt anyone—
intentionally.
It's a good goal
to speak impeccably
to avoid misunderstanding.
I'm imperfect,
and I understand words
hold the power of life and death.
I choose to speak life
because, with this awareness,
there's a possibility
of placing power where I can.
People's words have hurt me too.
I've seen people devastated by words
that put limits on their growth.

Don't let anyone limit
what's possible for you.
Don't let another human being
create a box around your life.
Use your words to free your soul.

Use everything to heal and grow;
your discernment will reveal the truth.
Become a master
of seeing the truth,
so you know what to let in
and what to leave behind.

GO BIG

When I stepped away
from certainty and stability,
I learned who I was
in uncertainty and instability.
I discovered the truth of who I was.
Both places are risky,
one keeps us the same
and the other challenges us deeply.
Growth happens
when we are pushed to confront
our limitations—
it shows us what we're made of.
I was given a choice—
to *go big* or *go home*.
The *going big*,
would test who I am,
going home showed me what I knew.
While being confronted with challenges,
I knew that going forward would build me
because the past could
no longer hold me.
I would fall
and get up stronger—
no matter what.

And in doing so,
I discovered there are always
open doors for me
when I let wisdom lead.

CONSCIOUS LIVING

For many people
pain has birthed their purpose—
experiencing hardships,
to become problem-solvers.
We need information from all sources
to understand the complexity of anything.
Everyone has a personal approach,
and it's only by looking at issues
in multiple ways
that we determine the truth.
Some are closer to the truth
and, ultimately,
the explanations will hit home
because they resonate within our souls.
Sometimes, at the beginning,
we may be so imbalanced
we can't see straight.
The right path will clear the confusion
and lead to more clarity.
With this process,
things improve fairly quickly.
The key is not to give up
but to keep searching for

the right alignment,
the right answers,
the right explanations.
In this way,
truth is ours,
and healing is too.

STEPPING STONES

No matter how bad it gets,
I want each of us to know
there's a way through—
to more knowledge and light.
We each have a consciousness
and a greater consciousness beyond us.
When we lack the answers,
seek more,
and we'll find more.
Everything is a hunt for the correct answers.
Sometimes, we're led to traps.
Sometimes, we're led to stepping stones.
Take the traps as fuel
to make more incredible leaps
on the stepping stones.
The truth is not shrouded
with manipulation.
Our soul knows when it's getting close.
Just listen to it
and be led to greater peace.

INNER GUIDANCE

Everyone we meet
has limits to their consciousness.
Everyone has different reasons
why they experience their challenges.
Each challenge is an opportunity
to unleash our superpowers.
Some of our superpowers
are in their infancy
and, with pressure,
we can reveal the best of ourselves.
When we feel the fire,
let it burn through our fears,
and ignite our magnificence.
Our challenges,
clearly show us,
we're made for more.
Nothing happens to us,
or for us—
in vain.

FREEDOM

If we listen to people
who tell us what's not possible—
we'll be lost.
We must be willing
to explore our imagination
of what's possible
and then create that environment
for ourselves.
Ignorance can stunt
any project from blossoming.
It's not noticeable initially,
but the impact is undeniable over time.
We'll wish we had opened our eyes sooner.
We'll wish we had walked away.
If we're honest with ourselves,
the correct knowledge
would have steered us
in a different direction.
When we finally see things
we couldn't see before,
let's be grateful—
it's our time
to move forward

muriel okubo

in a direction we choose
from a greater understanding.
Listen to our wisdom,
the truth in our souls.
We can live a fulfilled, honest life.

BUILDING

If we keep doing the right things,
we'll put the balance in our favour.
Making a house is the same—
building a solid foundation
often takes a long time,
and the rest moves relative to that.
When we have something good
to work with,
building can be fun.
We are our home.
We must create a foundation
and keep working at building it.
When we have a home,
we must maintain
and fix it when it needs mending—
getting to the problems quickly
and with diligence.
Don't ignore the signs of damage;
we can always restore them.
Nurture our home.
Listen to our home.
Support it when it needs more of this,
and less of that.

Keep it strong.
Keep the fires burning.
Keep caring for our home.

BEYOND THE SURFACE

When we're being tested
it'll feel like we're swimming
against the current,
gasping for air.
We'll feel like we aren't making progress,
and in those moments,
it's important to hold on and not panic.
Remain calm in the storm,
because those frightful moments will pass.
When it feels like our efforts
are returning in lack,
we're being given a spiritual hand,
and the divine is working through us,
providing power to places
that we can't touch.
It's crucial not to lose faith
when we can't see
what's happening.
It's like a body of water;
the surface often appears
smooth and cohesive,
but underneath,
there is a world of exciting activity
and networks that are divinely operating.

So let's do our best,
and surrender the rest.
Trust in this divinely designed life,
that holds all the secrets
that we don't know.

HEALERS

There are some people
who have lived through
excruciating turmoil,
and yet,
they can meet the pain of others.
They're the empaths of the world.
I have met incredible people
who have been healers on my path—
they're the ones who have compassion
that oozes from their being.
They're smart
but also wise.
They don't judge us in our presence
because they know
we're all one.
They've faced and slayed demons,
which is why they can meet us
to remind us that we can, too.
I'm grateful for the healers of the world.

PINCH ME

Patients will often be surprised
when they get well
because they're doubtful
of the enormous power we have.
They wonder if the results will last.
They tell me they don't want
to feel excited too soon,
fearing they'll jinx their results,
or that they might regress.
When we go through challenging times,
no one wants to return
to the scene of the crime.
The whole experience
holds a little PTSD.
We want to make sure,
we're well.
That it's all real.
Forever.
At the same time,
let's appreciate every day
we feel like ourselves
and keep humble
to this gift of life.

THE GIFT OF TODAY

We can heal.
We can be restored.
We can learn and become stronger.
We can use the opportunity before us
to be the best we can be.
We can see where we are and go from there.
This is all life is—
a chance to live it better each day.
Let go of the past.
Today is all we have.
All we need to do
is face it right now.

CALIBRATING

When something in your soul
tells you it isn't right,
keep going
until you make it right—
until everything is smooth again.
Learn to trust when
it's enough,
and when you need more.
You can recalibrate it all within yourself
every single day.
Be open to learning
and finding the balance—
the key to everything.
Choose to release what's too much
and receive only what you need.
All things
you know in your soul.

SOUL TRUTH

The truth is
you know more in your soul
than anyone on the planet—
scientists,
doctors,
researchers,
people who read the articles.
Truth is not in the lines,
nor in their minds,
nor in their souls.
You must be the one to determine
what to trust and to what degree.
The truth is in your soul.
Remember that the next time
they tell you what you should do
and what you shouldn't do.
The truth is in your soul.

THE POWER OF SURRENDER

Letting go was an exhaustive process
when I wasn't ready to let go of everything.
Sometimes, life will show us
what we must release to survive.
The habit of holding on can be heavy.
Sometimes, we don't get to
pick and choose what we get to keep.
In releasing it all,
I was birthed anew—
a change of pace, rhythm, and place.
Letting go and letting God
gave me the healing power to save my life.
It's by trusting a plan
that's larger than me—
orchestrated perfectly.
It's from here, I begin again;
to welcome new adventures,
to be free,
to enjoy the sun before it sets.
It's a trade-off with tremendous rewards.
There is divine wisdom guiding me,
and in surrendering,
I found freedom.
This is how I healed.

BABY STEPS

When we're held captive
to a force we can't control,
we must learn to focus
on what *we can* control.
What are the baby steps
we can manage at this moment?
What will make us feel okay right now?
What is good for our soul?
Our light is *ours*
no matter what darkness surrounds us.

FINE-TUNING

When thrown into chaos,
we must create organization to survive.
In chaos,
we'll discover a new playing ground
with new tricks to uncover.
This level has new rules,
none of which we've been privy to.
Being humble in the game,
we'll navigate the console of our lives,
with more flexibility
and grace for our mistakes.
It's easy to miss targets
and also be attacked,
when there's so much coming at us.
But when we play at levels
that demand more from us,
we'll find the best part of this whole thing,
is learning the instrument that is us.

LET GO

The best way to make ourselves
immune to the inequities
and traps of the world,
is by equipping ourselves with the truth,
and to allow everything else to pass on by.
The truth will embody divine love,
peace, health, and harmony.
In this approach,
we can be courageous
to ask for what we want,
seek the answers we have yet to see,
and to persist until a way opens.
As we subsist on goodness,
discerning what is not in alignment,
allows us to release with greater ease.
This is how we give ourselves ninety-nine lives.

UPGRADED

When your whole world
flips upside down,
you're set free
and given a chance
to walk upright again—
to know who you are,
to discover who you
truly came here to be.
In due time,
a whole new world emerges,
bringing clarity and peace.
Challenges have pushed you
to confront your boundaries
and expand your field.
Life has been reset for you,
to live more fully and deeply.
Life is not over for you
and you have more to give
to the world
and yourself.

CYCLE OF LIFE

Life is a continuous healing cycle—
you fall so you can learn to rise,
you lose so you can learn to win,
you fail so you can learn to succeed,
you have hardships
so you can learn to enjoy,
you have blocks,
so you can learn about freedom.
Rinse and repeat.
What a beautiful cycle.
And when you step outside the cycle,
you understand that every moment
is a gift for the next.

EYES TO SEE

The greatest thing we can do
is to derive understanding.
When we know how something works,
we can function better,
and don't need to suffer from confusion.
We can create a story to help ourselves
or we can create a story
that'll keep us stuck.
The future will unfold with grace
if we allow ourselves to live each moment
under the wing of wisdom.
Let's surrender to the truth
that is constantly being revealed to us.

FLUX

Life,
we start small
trying to get big
but come to realize big doesn't mean better.
Then we try to go back to being small.
It's in these adjustments we discover who we are
and where we fit.
Finding beauty in the blunders
and love in the darkness.
We're here to do it all one step at a time,
staying present in the wonder,
staying mindful of miracles,
and growing in the blessings of it all.

OPEN

I went on a fast
to clear the past—
it would be better than the last.
I had a blast,
less stuff to cast,
within me so vast.

JOY

In the trenches of pain,
I saw life in a
grand perspective.
This whole life
is a blessing—
the people I've met,
the roles I've played,
the things I've created,
the love I've experienced,
the laughs I've shared,
the miracles I've witnessed,
the growth in my being,
the gifts I've left,
the truth I've received,
the me that I am.
This is a whole life,
and I'm grateful for it all.

SPACE

When we can't rush time
nor control what comes next,
we can only face the moment.
In between breaths,
we discover
a piece of freedom.
It's a saving grace
from drowning
in the deep.
We learn to love our breath
because it offers us
a space to be.

FOCUS

Wherever you are today,
know your story
is not over yet.
You have memories to make,
more people to say I love you to,
dreams to live,
people to be loved by,
and moments to enjoy.
Use the fire in your soul
to lead you today.
Do what you must do today.
Every day will be different.
Tomorrow's a new day.
Breathe, knowing you only
must worry about today.

YOUR STORY

I have learned
the only way
to get through life
in one piece
is by giving it meaning,
and only we
can do this for ourselves.
When darkness is all we see,
give it a story as dynamic as the ocean,
it will transform and dazzle us,
and remind us of the beauty and power
found only in the beholder.

SAVORING

I don't doubt
there are angels in our lives.
I've met some of them.
They push me to be my best.
They allow me to be me,
while also reminding me of parts,
I've forgotten.
I find joy in all this,
because we never know
when our chances here
end.

PRESENCE

No one has the complete truth—
our knowledge is incomplete.
When we die,
we'll get it all—
the complete picture.
Until then,
have faith
that the rest of our lives holds
better days
and the best unfolds
when we focus on today.

HOLD ON

Life moves fast.
In trying times,
it feels torturously slow.
No one can tell you
what the future holds,
but your soul knows
it wants you to soar.
It believes in you
and your desire
to move forward
and cheers for you to envision
a bright future
as assured as the sun.

BREAD OF LIFE

When we don't have many needs,
life is easy.
And when we lack what we need,
life can be tricky.
Our bodies will seek to survive first,
and luxuries no longer matter.
Love provides us
with sustenance
when we have lost our life raft.
Love still gives
when there is nothing left.

THAWING

Everything feels like a dark, snowy,
windy winter night on the prairies,
when you face your humanity.
Like being thrown out in the cold
with nowhere to go.
Nowhere to find shelter
when the places you used to go
are taken away from you—
comfort zones,
familiar haunts,
mind-numbing movies,
play-time—
all taken away
because all you have time for is
keeping your toes, fingers, and nose
from freezing.
And life can change in an instant,
when someone opens the door
and warms you with their light,
life begins to flow again.

ALL IN

People often say
God doesn't give us
more than we can handle.
When our limits are tested,
we pray that nothing
will ever go that far again.
When death makes its presence known,
we realize how much we love life,
and we begin to discover
the strength to build a fire
to burn through the mess.
We don't want to take the scenic route,
but a direct flight—
through the blocks,
the pain,
and the suffocation.
We're not leaving anything for later.
We'll give it all we have
because our lives are precious.

NO FLUFF

I never had a chance to fear,
because I was on a mission
to restore myself.
Like when we don't have time
or energy to waste on things
that brings us down.
I became good at compartmentalizing
my energy and time.
What would give me the most relief?
My purpose was only to find solace.
Thankfully,
long ago,
I knew the value of holding focus
and would not let anything deter me.
I had a laser-like vision
of where I needed to go,
and this is what saved my life.

DELIVERY

Dear You,
I believe you're here for a reason,
and you might not know it yet,
but people's lives are blessed
because you exist.
Your life has a purpose,
and your job is to decode what that is.
Your soul won't stop tugging at your heart
until you pursue the path
it longs for.

REVELATION

I speak a lot about love
because I know it intimately.
It's the only place I feel at home.
I won't make a home
anyplace else
anymore.
When we begin to see,
we can't unsee ever again.

I'M LISTENING

When feelings and memories
hit us from time to time,
we'll get a little weepy.
We must let ourselves feel them again
because there's a story they need to tell us.
It's often a beautiful message,
the inner divine in us
will always have our back,
no matter what we face.
We send a thank you
to the one who created our souls.

OCEAN

When we've been restored
from something that rocks our world,
gratitude becomes our most significant truth.
We're left to make meaning
of everything that happened,
because no one can understand it
the way we do.
The gravity of situations is our gift—
to be used to ground us
when we have no words to explain
the tsunami of everything we experienced.
We want to save the world
from all that hurt us,
but sometimes we must wait
to make sure another tide
will not sweep us away.
This is what it's like
when we've found our breath
after we've been swallowed.

TRAINING

When the ground cradles you
when you've hit rock bottom,
you'll discover a wisdom that
can only come from humbling yourself
to that level.
When you embrace the stillness,
it has much to teach you.
You gain more understanding
of humility,
of surrender,
of honesty,
of nakedness.
It would be from this place,
you would also find the strength
to build,
take charge,
be authentic,
and put on your armour
to rise to fight again.

NO WINNERS

There is a war against our health
and I was born into it.
I've seen miracles
despite all the tragedies.
I've seen tragedies
despite all the miracles.
I don't know
who wins this war.
I'm sure it takes many victims
while the valiant keep trying.
I don't think wars
leave any winners.
Troubled souls roam this earth
ignorant of honour and love.
Some have chosen to play the game
with no integrity.
We all continue to lose
if we don't stand together
and discover the love
that is bound in our souls.

ON FIRE

Everyday,
is a choice to grab that morsel
of strength and to direct it with fire
toward your healing and restoration.
Don't let anyone or anything
distract you,
or put out your fire.
Know with certainty
that you aren't meant to stay
in a forever season of pain.
Use your fire
to be on fire
for your life.

EXPANSION

When you feel there's something
not quite right with yourself—
you're right.
You need not prove that
to anyone else.
The truth is in your soul.
Find people who understand your hardship
and don't pass judgement
on your observations.
We all need help sometimes,
and the people
who appreciate your astuteness
will be your cheerleaders.
Your expansion will lead
to their expansion.
Trust in the truth of what you know.

IT'S NOT OVER

Life threw me a curveball,
and I would play my part
with all my might.
We each have a life force
that wants us to hit it
out of the park.
I'm rooting for everyone
who needs to heal,
who feels things are too heavy to carry.
Just keep showing up,
and don't give up
till' every last ounce of our being
is left out on the field.

EARTH SCHOOL

The truth is embedded in our souls.
The lessons we need to learn
put us exactly where we need to be.
Although life's tough,
I know we're more powerful
than anything we face.
Everything allows us
to become wiser
and more discerning,
if we humbly allow
ourselves to be schooled.

THE GIFT OF CHANGE

I have been blessed
to see people heal.
It's the lens
through which I see.
I don't doubt,
because I know
one small shift
can change it all.
This is a gift for you and me.

GENTLE PEACE

I sat as the sun rose today,
and the fresh air filled my soul—
the beautiful colours I can see.
I sip my cup of green tea.
In the quiet and stillness,
health never felt so good.
It isn't the crazy stuff
we miss when life's in chaos.
It's the simple peace
we miss the most.

HEART HAVEN

When you're sick,
who do you go to?
These are the people
who love and understand you.
You don't have to hide
how fragile you are.
You don't have to be afraid
to be seen by them
even when you feel
like a stranger to your soul.
Bless these souls who care
for you with compassion and kindness
and leave judgment at the door.
Thank you to these souls
who provide shelter in storms.

HOME

I know love heals,
because I've witnessed it
in my own life,
and in the lives of others.
If we find ourselves in a dark place,
seek someone who will listen
and be soft and patient.
When everything feels like a jagged edge,
it's in the round, kind places
that our souls can rest and heal.
Our heart will find peace
in spiritual comfort.

MUSTARD SEED

I know people are strong.
They tell me incredible things
and all they've overcome in their lives.
Some people endure the wildest things,
yet they're here to share their stories.
We are unique and special,
and when one person survives
to tell their story,
it inspires another person
to believe in possibility—
to have faith in the power inside
all of us.

FORGIVING YOURSELF

It's easy to be disappointed in ourselves
because of the things we couldn't perceive,
or the things we didn't know how to
approach.
We can't judge the consciousness
we had at that time,
because our consciousness grows
usually after it happens.
This wisdom is our gift
for moving through the waves of life
and embracing and accepting ourselves
regardless of the pain it caused.
If we learn,
it served its purpose.

THE SERVICE OF LOVE

When we realize that lacking knowledge
can hurt us in this world,
it's a tough place to be.
We fall into traps
that we must dig ourselves out of.
In the process,
we learn monumental lessons.
Life will humble us
because it wants us
to derive truth from our experiences.
The most significant gift
comes from sharing what we know
with those who seek solace from us.
Then, our purpose will be
to learn and expand more.
The key is remaining open
to the things that challenge us
and not to shut down when
life wounds us.
Love is the answer to all our woes.
Like a miracle, love heals.

MIND RENEWAL

We all make "mis-" "takes,"
lacking clarity and judgement
in moments of limited consciousness.
Our mistakes can hurt us,
but there's also grace
that understands our intentions.
We're human,
and it's our mistakes that help
to refine, strengthen, and purify us.
The next time
we make a mistake,
we can recognize the part of us
that's striving to grow.
Often, we need these reminders
to be careful as we create
a future with more clarity.
Take time to gain perspective
and use the knowledge
we've gained
to craft a better vision.

NO LIMITS

The more we learn,
the more we know,
the more we grow,
the more we can be of service,
the more we can appreciate,
the more we can forgive,
the more we love,
the more we believe,
the more we receive.

BLESSED

It's the kind souls
I've encountered
who have helped heal me the most.
They've listened, respected,
and cared for me,
when the ground had fallen away.
I thank God for those who had
arms to hug me,
the patience to sit with me,
the gentleness to cry with me,
the strength to endure with me,
the safety to let me unravel,
the kindness to see my heart,
the love to witness my soul.
These are the people
with whom God blessed my path
to remind me
I'm loved,
and never alone.

GROWTH

We open our ears to listen more,
We open our eyes to see more,
We open our hearts to feel more,
We open our soul to receive more.
In becoming humble in this life,
we understand how limited,
we've been to the limitless.

FREE FLOW

In some moments,
we'll feel strong,
and in some moments,
we'll feel weak.
Some moments feel like
they'll last forever
and some don't last long enough.
This is the transience of life.
This information is for us
to discover what brings life
and what takes it away.
Only we can decide what to take in
and what to leave behind.
If we can appreciate everything
we've been blessed with,
then, naturally,
the moments of grace will last longer
and spill into all the moments of our lives.
This is how light overcomes darkness.

EMPOWERMENT

Change your perspective.
What can you do
with the information you have?
You get to choose the story.
Will this event encourage
you to soar and make positive changes,
or will it crumble you?
The divine power within you
is not extinguishable.
It's your gift to move this power
in the direction of your choice.
Your mind might tell you that
you can't get over what happened,
but events don't hold power—
you do.
Take the lessons,
and approach life as though
your next moment is a gift
to change it in your favour.
What moves your life in a way
that holds kindness, love, and truth?
Choose to be the hero in your own story.

YOUR STORY

You fall.
You get up.
You fall.
You get up.
You fall.
You get up.
You fall.
You get up.
You fall.
You get up.
You fall.
You get up.
You fall.
You get up.
The moral of this story:
you'll get up
every time you fall.
You won't stay down.

KINDNESS

Kindness is something
we all have—
and we often forget
its simple power.
Remember its essence
on your most challenging days.
Kindness is saying something
you think they already know.
Kindness is doing something
just because you love them.
Kindness is the intention
in the words you don't say.
Kindness is the warmth
that thaws you after losing everything.
Kindness is the gift you give
when you have nothing to gain.
Kindness will heal the souls
who come into your life
seeking respite
from the world's darkness.
Keep kindness in your light.

SOUL CALL

Our soul will hold us here
as long as it can
to help us to learn the lessons
we need to know.
Every day is an opportunity
to use this lifeline,
to live our lives
in a way we're proud of—
with integrity and grace.
When our mind, body, and soul
operate as one,
it's a glimpse of being alignment
with our soul.

RESTORED

When we survive one challenge,
and the next one
is right in front of us,
it means we have
more strength than we know.
It's a reminder
we're going through a growth spurt
and to embrace change.
Life ebbs and flows,
and it nudges us to breathe through it all.
Our breath will create space
in the present moment
and make our expansion
graceful and elevating.
We'll discover
day by day,
moment by moment,
more bits of sunshine that peak through.
As we take in these moments,
we'll unveil a grin,
a smile,
a laugh.
These are all we need to let our hearts
come back to love.

FOR IT TO BE SO

In the process of healing,
faith is the most important thing you have.
It'll lift you on days
that you don't think you can make it,
and it'll give you just enough strength
to believe in the things you don't see
or experience yet.
Take hold of faith every moment
you think you're too small
to defeat your dragons.
Slowly, this attitude will bring you
to a new level.
Faith will always bring new light
in times of darkness.
Faith will birth your miracle.

NOT GIVING IN

If you keep trying,
there's no way to fail.
There might be detours,
and steps backward,
but it's these shifts,
that eventually propel you forward.
Sometimes, you don't know what's working
unless you win sometimes,
and lose sometimes.
Apply your efforts to what works,
and you will make sudden leaps.
Always remember
that tweaking is your superpower.
Self-awareness is the only way
to overcome the hurdles to greater health.

FOCUSED DIRECTION

When things happen
outside of your control,
it will make you feel
vulnerable and weak.
In these times,
give yourself compassion,
and remind yourself of the power
you do have.
What's in your control,
is more than enough,
to conquer this overwhelming beast
that you face.
Your power,
is in the way you direct your thoughts,
the people you choose to be around,
holding the attitude of a victor,
and moving in the direction of health
every moment that you're blessed with.

BEYOND YOURSELF

When life confronts you
and you can't calmly pass over it,
it's giving you a chance
to see the precious child inside of you,
who is relying on you to make things right.
It's honouring the little person inside of you,
who begs you for their life—
to fight with everything you have,
to save them too.
With more wisdom
and courage than ever before,
you'll meet your soul
face to face
and surrender completely.
This is the moment,
that leads you to your breakthrough,
because you aren't going to let them down.
You're going to find the courage
to make a way
for both of you.

BRAND NEW

You'll need to stop comparing
the you before this,
and the you after this.
You've changed.
Give yourself permission
to be something new.
Give yourself permission
to be different.
Heal in the way
your new self needs,
not in the way your old self would have.
It's okay that you have nowhere to return to,
but the path boldly before you.
What's freeing and renewing healed you,
and this is what your brain, body, and spirit
need right now.

DEATH AND BIRTH

In many ways,
we're dying from the start
and being born again.
Our cells are constantly changing—
growing, repairing, and dying.
This is something to be grateful for—
the ability to know
we can transform.
We can come back better than we were—
stronger,
clearer,
wiser.
More us.
And this happens
to all our cells—
the tiniest minutia of us.
We can release the past
and all the toxicity.
We can let go of what isn't divine
and embrace all that is.
This is the gift of life.

PURPOSE

When life flashes before your eyes,
you'll find that you're grateful for everything.
You're grateful that your soul touched
everything that made it dance and be free.
You're happy to have met amazing people.
Every challenge in your life
has accentuated
your attitude of gratitude.
You know what it's like
to feel invincible,
and you know what it's like
to feel vulnerable.
Not a day passes
when you cease to say thank you
for where you are today.
You may have sacrificed a lot of things,
but you have your life
and, for that,
you feel blessed.

IN THE MIDST

On the path of healing,
you'll wonder
when you'll feel like yourself again.
These physical challenges and tests
will encourage you to strengthen and develop
your spiritual power—
the place where prayers are answered,
cries are heard,
blindness cured,
and hope is transformed.
Your spirit is what drives your physical self,
and when pushed beyond
what's in your control,
the spiritual world will feel closer than
any place you've been.
Your spirit is the heartbeat behind
everything you do—
your thoughts, choices, actions, and willpower.
Tend to your spirit with love,
and your next steps
will birth your physical miracles.

THE GREAT DIVIDE

The more I understand
the world's inequities,
the deeper they get.
There are many dark parts,
and many light parts too.
When I see great pain,
I'm also aware there is great love.
We all must make our way through life,
navigating the light and the dark.
And at the end,
yin and yang separate,
and our souls are set free
for the next adventure.
I choose to stay with the side
of love.

WAKING UP

When the world you know has changed,
it won't feel ephemeral
but something that will hit you hard.
You have been through hard times,
but the magnitude will be different.
You'll have to move with intuition
instead of what's familiar.
When you have nothing to fall back on,
falling forward is the only way.
There is no other way to freedom.

DODGING LANDMINES

Some battles can't be fought
while you're sick on the battlefield
praying for peace.
All you can do
is put your energy
into regaining your strength
and your will to survive.
It's enough—
to see another day,
when you're fighting for your life.
All the fight must go into you,
when energy is precious and scarce.
With finite energy,
there's no time to spend on futile missions,
finding blaming for your plight.
Your best will come by
giving yourself everything you have.

EMBRACING UNCERTAINTY

Sometimes you won't know
what you're capable of,
unless you're put into a situation,
that tests every fibre of your being.
And it'll exhaust you,
but you must constantly
feed your mind with hope.
If you choose to see your life
as a possibility versus an impasse,
you'll find the breakthrough
to overcome your blocks.

REST, BUT DON'T QUIT

Don't stop
until you get the results
that give you peace.
There's a reason
you're restless;
because you can't rest without
the one hundred percent that you deserve.
Health is one of those things,
you must demand for yourself.
Trust in the healing capacity
of this brilliantly designed system.
The only thing that stops total healing
is something we don't understand.
Take it one day at a time,
and seek to increase your knowledge
to move you closer to the truth—
the place of your wholeness.

LET THE LIGHT LEAD YOU

The miracle you need is just a shift away;
a focus of light in the right direction—
a heavy head down shifted towards the sky,
a smile when you want to frown,
a laugh amid of a cry,
a rabbit hole that leads you to the truth,
a person's story of overcoming,
a hug that breaks your fall,
a blog that details a remedy,
a walk that inspires you,
a loved one who loves you.
Use these bits of light to shift you
out of the darkness into the light.
These are the glimpses of your healing
and restoration.
Keep going.

TRUTH HEALS

Don't settle for lies.
The world is rampant with them.
We've been exposed to many of them
that have been normalized
and disguised as the truth.
The truth frees us,
and lies hurt us.
If we're hurting,
it's our job to seek the truth,
and free ourselves.
This is part of the journey of our lives here.

WHOLENESS

Wholeness is aligning
with our divine nature;
the truth of our completeness,
our supernatural healing powers,
knowing we have access to wisdom,
letting love lead us,
and living in harmonious ways.

NO OTHER OPTIONS

Restoration is possible.
and your healing is too.
Don't succumb to fear
when it sets its traps everywhere.
Move away from the thoughts that tell you
you can't make it,
you're not strong enough,
or it's too painful.
If you focus on your restoration,
there's no room to entertain
anything else.

HEALING THE ROOT

Finding what causes you to suffer,
will allow you to overcome it.
When you understand what afflicts you,
you can start to determine
how to remove them.
When you know what you're dealing with,
you can use the right tools,
and methods,
to break free.

HEALTH RIGHTS

You're meant to heal.
You're meant to thrive.
You're meant to be well.
Don't believe any lies
that whisper to you of anything contrary.
Do what a person who is healed;
would do.
Do what a person who is thriving;
would do.
Do what a person who is well;
would do.
Do what a person who knows
that this is not the end;
would do.
This is how you turn the tables,
and align with your destiny of health.

LEAN IN

Find strength from good people
who will share their kindness
when you need it,
who help build up your reserves,
supporting you to stand again.
They'll feed your spirit,
when you're barely hanging on.
Remember it's okay
to seek support when facing
the greatest war of your life.
Regain your power,
with those who remind you
of your strength.

GROWING PAINS

The path to healing often goes in waves
while still following an upward trajectory.
There will be times
when your emotions will fluctuate,
from hopeful to frustrated,
but when you feel terrible,
that's the time to push through.
These dips are a sign to keep moving
through the pain—
often, your next-level advancement
is on the other side of pressing through
these heart-breaking episodes.
In the big picture,
progress is being made,
but your emotions only see
black and white—
healed or not healed yet.
Let yourself observe and feel your feelings,
without judgement.
When you return to a state of calm,
allow yourself to appreciate
the truth of your progress.

WHOLE YOU

Wholeness will feel a little surreal
when you haven't had peace
for a long time.
Embrace and be excited for every moment,
that life feels like you again.
There's nothing like health
and nothing better than it.

ONE-TRACK MIND

Become a priority to yourself.
Humbly listen to your inner being.
Understand what's being called of you;
find the knowledge
and support you need
to uncover the peace you're craving.
Answers will be revealed
in the most extraordinary ways
as you focus your intention.
You'll expose solutions and ideas
that will seep into your consciousness.
The truth is out there,
to support your healing,
when you have a one-track mind
to destination wholeness.

NEVER GIVE UP

While returning yourself to good health,
never throw in the towel.
It's like in a game;
your opponent
taunts you to say, "give."
With every breath,
you can change the tide
in your favour.
It's in giving up
that everything's lost.
It doesn't matter where you end up,
as long as you make do
with what's in front of you.
This present moment is where it counts.
You can't fail by giving it your all.
Looking back,
this is how you made it through.

THANK YOU FOR PURCHASING RESTORED TO WHOLENESS

Thank you very much for purchasing my book. I hope this book comforts and encourages your heart, spirit and soul. Sometimes, the right words can give you what you need to feel understood and endure your most challenging days. I pray for your complete healing and restoration.

If you've found Restored to Wholeness to be a source of inspiration and value, I'd love for you to share your thoughts in a review. Your feedback is greatly appreciated. Thank you once again!

Warmly,

Muriel Okubo

SUBSCRIBE TO MY NEWSLETTER

Find me on my website: okubowellness.com
Follow me on IG: @muriel.okubo @okubowellness

ABOUT THE AUTHOR

Muriel Okubo is a Canadian-Japanese author, artist, and Doctor of Traditional Asian Medicine. She has had a busy practice for over sixteen years in which she has treated people from all walks of life and all ages struggling with various issues. Having witnessed the pains of the human condition and the beauty of the human spirit, she wishes to inspire and encourage everyone on their path.

Understanding that body-mind-spirit health is crucial for wellness, she has created beautiful books to help people integrate their physical, mental, emotional, and spiritual bodies. She has always loved the power of writing as a connection to her heart and soul. Muriel is passionate about sharing the ideas and practices that have helped her the most on her path to living more consciously. She desires that everyone follow their inner wisdom and find the truth of their soul.